MW01714211

Voices of Resilience

Breast Cancer Survivor Narratives from the Mohawk Valley

Voices of Resilience

Breast Cancer Survivor Narratives from the Mohawk Valley

Joanne Joseph, Ph.D.
Patricia Murphy, D.A.

Nicholas K. Burns Publishing
Utica, New York

Nicholas K. Burns Publishing
130 Proctor Boulevard
Utica, New York 13501
www.nkbpublishing.com

Printed in the United States of America
ISBN 13: 978-0-9755224-4-8

Cover photo and book and cover design by Lynne Browne

Library of Congress Control Number: 2009928131

Dedication

I would like to dedicate this book to breast cancer survivor Cindy Haddon, whose spirit and determination have been an example for my life throughout many years of friendship, even over the many miles that separate us.

– *Patricia Murphy*

Some people impact your life at a time when their struggles are the greatest. This was certainly the case for my mother, Louise Joseph, and my good friend, Kathy Britton. Both women faced the challenge of breast cancer with courage, hope, and fortitude. Their lives and their struggles with breast cancer show just how resilient the human spirit really is. This book is dedicated to them and to the other resilient men and women who inspire us to hope and persevere in the face of adversity.

– *Joanne Joseph*

Contents

Preface

Patricia Murphy, D. A.

This book is the result of a service-learning writing project at the SUNY Institute of Technology in Utica, New York. These are real people's stories, and gathering them meant exposing students to a different educational model, service-learning. Service-learning has many different definitions and can take many forms, but at its crux is the belief that students can learn through interactions with people outside of their campus communities as much as they can learn from classroom experiences. Implementing the project meant taking a chance that students would connect with our community participants and learn from them. Importantly, believing in a project like this one means recognizing and valuing the power of narratives.

Narratives are stories. They are the family tales we tell each other over and over again when we want to be reassured that we have a connection to and history with other people. Narratives can be a way to share knowledge and to create new knowledge. Narratives are an important part of our lives because they allow us to remember events and people after our original experiences are over. Using narrative, we can revisit memories so that we won't forget how important they are. When we tell our stories, we also pass down our emotional responses to events, and that infusion of emotion is as important as getting the details "right." From the emotional content of our stories, our listeners and readers can understand so much.

The service-learning project from which this book came has as its theoretical basis an idea about the value that lies in talking to others and learning about them in order to connect to the world at large. As a writing teacher, one of my goals is to help students on a journey of changing perception. Traditional (those right out of high school) students come to college at a developmental stage, at a time in their lives, when they are starting to see themselves as more than center and more than periphery in their relationship to the world at large. Composition and citizenry are considered to go hand-in-hand because the critical thinking and exchange of ideas that occurs in the classroom is exemplary of (and practice for) the way we become citizens. So as a composition teacher, I have to theorize and implement ways to get students to think about two worlds—the world of college and the world beyond—and I have to show students, too, that those worlds are not so different or separate as they sometimes think.

Narrative was used twice in the service-learning

composition class that became the basis for this book. First, students wrote a first person narrative discussing an encounter with illness, either a firsthand illness or one experienced by someone to whom they were close. Later in the course, students read articles that discussed the value of illness narratives as they interviewed the women whose stories are contained in the book. The question they wanted to answer was what value does telling illness narratives have for narrators and listeners?

The idea of empowerment is important to the project. I wanted my students to feel empowered by their encounters with our respondents, and I wanted the respondents to feel that talking to my students empowered them. Again, there is the simple belief that the power of storytelling can have great impact on tellers and listeners. My hope was that my students would emerge from this project feeling like they could overcome obstacles because they had made a connection with people who had overcome so much.

So three strands, a belief that acts of service enhance a college education, a belief in narrative as a way of getting students involved in their education, and a belief in the emotional and psychological power of narrative come together in this book. The students who participated in the project showed genuine interests in the stories told to them by the respondents. They recognized resilient traits in the respondents and concluded that telling illness narratives can contribute positively to the overall experience of cancer treatment and recovery. Many students commented that they were surprised at how vibrant the respondents were, testimony to the strides this project made toward reducing negative stereotypes associated with serious illness.

One student wrote:

> So why do these people take the time out of their schedules to share their stories with us? Because, in its own way, it's therapeutic. Medicine and science can only do so much to better the body, but telling their stories is a way of bettering their minds, emotions, and spirit. These people fought against the odds and proved the doubters wrong . . . Stories help the narrator and audience in different ways. The story helped the narrator, because she showed through her expressions that she was very proud of her accomplishments. As she tells her story, she can remind herself of how far she has gone in her recovery and that she can continue to improve herself in the future. I was also affected by the narrator's story. When you get a first person point of view, you can better understand how to help people in these types of situations.

This typical example indicates that the student recognized the value of interviewing the respondent and learning about illness narratives.

Of course, this book would not be possible without the generous women whose stories are told within. Members of the After Breast Cancer Support Network (ABC) group and non members alike gave up their time to talk to students and teachers candidly about their illness experiences. The subjects they covered range from medical and family relationships to chemotherapy, surgical, and radiation treatments, from the physical aspects of cancer to the importance of humor and determination.

While converting interviews to essays and revising and editing their texts, I tried to do more than get the facts straight; I tried to preserve their individual voices so that readers could understand what it felt like for these women to face breast cancer. Their strength and generosity was almost overwhelming at times. The time they took to talk to my students meant that we could all share an insightful and memorable experience. Although the women whose stories make up this book come from different backgrounds and places, one thing can be said of all of them: They are gifted storytellers and profound role models for us all.

Acknowledgments

The authors wish to thank:

The members of the After Breast Cancer Support Network (ABC), Utica, New York for sharing their stories.

The SUNYIT students who participated in this project.

John Snizek of Crystal Springs Golf Course, Vernon, New York and the Golfing for Breast Cancer committee for funding this project.

Lynne Browne for formatting this text, designing the cover, and for sharing her story.

Karen Christensen for starting the After Breast Cancer Support Network and for sharing her story.

Maureen Cool for transcribing interviews in this book.

The State University of New York Institute of Technology for its support.

Suzanne Burns, RN, of the Comprehensive Breast Care Center at Faxton-St. Luke's Healthcare in Utica, New York for all of her help.

Introduction

Breast Cancer, Resilience and Post-Traumatic Growth

Joanne Joseph, Ph.D.

Talk to most women and they will tell you that the thought of having breast cancer is frightening, even though treatment strategies and outcomes have improved over the years. It is not surprising, therefore, that feelings of anxiety and depression often accompany a diagnosis of breast cancer (Stanton and Snyder 1993).

However, many breast cancer patients adjust well to the diagnosis. Some are even able to grow personally from the experience. Psychologists refer to this satisfactory adjustment to breast cancer as positive adaptation or resilience (Bonanno 2004). They refer to the ability to grow from the experience as "post-traumatic growth" (Tedeschi and Kilmer 2005).

What accounts for resilience and post-traumatic growth? Both result from personal traits and what resilience researchers call "protective factors" in the environment (Masten 2004). This book illustrates both the personal traits and protective factors present in a resilient breast cancer survivor. Let's take a look at those personal traits and protective factors in greater detail.

Personal Traits

Researchers have identified a number of personal traits associated with positive adaptation and resilience. These traits include:

1. A tendency to be **proactive** rather than reactive. In the case of breast cancer, this means taking charge of your situation. This is in contrast to waiting for someone else to make all the decisions or reacting negatively to situations that you cannot control. Good examples of "take charge" or proactive traits include seeking out information and support, choosing your health care team, and planning for treatment complications. The proactive approach to problem solving for breast cancer survivors requires balancing self-reliance and independence with the willingness to recognize and accept help from others.

2. **Self-efficacy** means that you believe you have the ability and resources to effectively manage your care and course of treatment. Self-efficacy demands an understanding of the resources available to you, what your needs are, and what plan of action will best suit you as you navigate through treatment.

3. A **sense of challenge** and an **optimistic outlook**. People with a challenge-orientation extract

opportunity out of adversity. In the case of breast cancer, this means using the breast cancer in a way that might benefit you or others. There are several excellent examples of the challenge orientation in the stories that follow.

We commonly define optimism as the general belief that good outcomes will occur in the future. People who are more optimistic tend to have better outcomes even when they are not overly realistic (Taylor 2008). A sense of challenge and an optimistic perspective are two of the most important resiliency traits.

4. People deal with adversity more effectively when they have **goals** or reasons for persevering. Goals make the negative aspects of therapy easier to deal with. They also fuel the person's motivation to recover and grow from the experience. Often the goals relate to the needs of other people. For example, it is common for individuals to persevere in the face of threatening illness for the sake of children or significant others.

   In effect, concern for others becomes the reason for sticking with treatments like chemotherapy or radiation even though the side effects might be difficult to tolerate at times.

5. The ability to bring some **meaning and purpose** to the experience. Dealing with a stressful event like breast cancer often prompts people to think about

their lives in a different way. This trait is a common theme in our narratives. Essentially, the women in this book thought about the cancer as a catalyst for change. They believe that because they had cancer, they are better people. Or, because of the cancer, they developed a new appreciation of life. These realizations are examples of how people bring meaning to their cancer experience.

Research tells us that people adapt better to difficult situations when they apply purpose to them (Vickberg, Bovbjerg, DuHamel, Currie, and Redd 2000). Examples in the book are patients who believe breast cancer helped them become better people, and breast cancer survivors who use their spirituality to deal with the diagnosis.

Protective Factors

Researchers studying resilient breast cancer survivors have identified a number of protective factors. The narratives that follow highlight two of those factors: hearing stories from other survivors and social support from other people in the individual's life.

Hearing the stories of other women who have had the experience is often satisfying and helpful (Taylor 2008). This is because stories provide the breast cancer survivor with relevant information about treatment and the opportunity to connect with real people who have been through the experience.

Information is a powerful tool. Information about breast cancer treatment minimizes the mystery and uncertainty of the treatment regimen. It contributes to a person's proactive attitude and sense of self-efficacy because it allows the person to anticipate and plan for treatment. A number of the stories in this book speak to the power of information and knowledge. Many of the women whose stories are contained within these pages actively sought out information about their breast cancer and the treatment options open to them. Their reports mirror the research findings of many others, verifying the psychological benefits of information (Taylor 2008).

Stories about other people with similar experiences provide examples or models for breast cancer patients. Narratives tell the breast cancer story from a breast cancer survivor's point of view. People are naturally attracted to others who have experienced what they are about to experience, especially if that experience is negative or novel (Kugaya and Okamura 2001, Pennebaker and Seagal 1999).

They use the people in the story as models or guides for what to expect and how to behave. These stories can be and often are a source of hope and support for those first confronted with the diagnosis (Frank 1997). A number of the women in this book sought out others to talk to about the experience, and their reactions to these narratives were helpful and instructive.

Like good stories, social supports are essential for resilience and post-traumatic growth. Social supports come in several forms. For example, there are expert, emotional, and instrumental social supports. Health care professionals who are willing to discuss treatment options and family and friends who offer assistance and are just willing to listen are examples of social support.

Social support is powerful. Researchers find that social support significantly predicts the quality and sometimes the quantity of life a person will have. Those with good social supports live better with their cancer than those who do not have a support system in place (Taylor 2008). This is because social support provides people with the resources they need during a crisis. It also provides an important sense of connection that helps when you feel vulnerable, especially when first diagnosed with breast cancer.

We designed this collection to tell the story of thirteen remarkable women. Their narratives reinforce the fact that people can not only survive the experience of breast cancer, but can also grow from the experience. Each of the stories is a unique example of the resilient traits and factors mentioned above. These stories provide wonderful lessons about how to deal with breast cancer and the consequences of treatment. Each of the stories underscores the importance of social support and the resilience of the human spirit. We will be eternally grateful to all the women who contributed to this book. Enjoy!

References

Bonanno, G.A. (2004). Loss, trauma, and human resilience: Have we underestimated the human capacity to thrive after extremely aversive events? *American Psychologist,* 59(1), 20-28.

Frank, A.W. (1997). *The Wounded Storyteller.* Chicago: University of Chicago Press

Kugaya, F.S., Okamura, H. (2001). Psychosocial group intervention and breast cancer. *Evidence-Based Mental Health,*4, 15.

Masten, A. S. (2001). Ordinary magic: Resilience process in development. *American Psychologist,* 56(3), 227-238.

Pennebaker, J.W., Seagal, J.D. (1999). Forming a story: The health benefits of narrative. *Journal of Clinical Psychology,* 55(10), 1243-1254.

Stanton, A.L., Snider (1993). Coping with a breast cancer diagnosis: A prospective study. *Health Psychology,* 12 (1) 16-23.

Taylor, S. E. (2008). Health Psychology. Boston: McGraw Hill.

Tedeschi, R.G; Kilmer, R.P. (2005). Assessing strengths, resilience, and growth to guide clinical Interventions. Professional Psychology: Research and Practice, 36(3), 230-237.

Vickberg, S.M.J.; Bovbjerg, D.H.;DuHamelK.N.;Currie, V.; Redd, W.H. (2000). Intrusive thoughts and psycholgical distress among breast cancer survivors: Global meaning as a possible protective factor. Behavioral Medicine, 25, 152-160.

One

Karen

I was born in 1941 in Utica and raised in Marcy, New York, the younger of two children, the only girl. I graduated college majoring in Advertising, Design and Production. But, for whatever reason, in 1963 life's path led me to occupational therapy at a psychiatric center. I took additional courses to become an art therapist. This was probably the first time that I realized I loved working with people. In 1986 my life took another turn.

My particular story is not heroic or inspirational. I had a routine mammogram which proved positive for breast cancer. It came as a shock, which it does to all of us. Twenty-two years ago I was a runner, didn't eat red meat, I was much thinner, I had given up smoking seven years previous to that, and had no history of breast cancer in my family. I never read any of the women's magazines with breast cancer articles because I had no reason to think I'd ever get this disease. There were only a few articles because there was not a lot of hoopla in 1986 about breast cancer. No pink ribbons, no breast cancer walks or particular emphasis on the disease. I really knew nothing about breast cancer.

For the first few days I was numb with fear. I felt I needed to be familiar with the sound of, *"I have breast cancer,"* so I wrote letters to friends who lived out of state only so I could see the words in print... *"I have breast cancer."* There were no specific support groups to turn to, and the few women I knew who had breast cancer had succumbed to the disease.

I sought the opinions of two doctors; both suggested that I have a mastectomy. Things happen in a sort of fast/slow-motion way when you are threatened by a life altering disease. Every single woman who has faced a diagnosis of breast cancer will tell you her life changes on the day the doctor says "you have breast cancer." That doesn't mean it changes for the worst, but at that moment you probably think it's the worst. Once you get some distance from your diagnosis you realize you've gained strengths that you never knew you had.

Looking back, I am always amazed that I was able to negotiate my way through that terrifying cancer jungle. Cancer doesn't choose where it occurs in your life; it happens no matter what you are doing, whether you are at your happiest moment in life or at a time when you are overcome with personal problems.

I quickly learned that if I did one thing at a time and stayed away from the "what ifs" I did better. For example, there was a time I dreaded being fifty, then suddenly I realized, *"what if"* I don't live to see fifty! Cancer does have a way of putting things into perspective! Immediately after a diagnosis there is a natural tendency to see only the dark clouds, when in fact there really is a blue sky background behind those clouds.

My sense of humor has always guided my life. I love laughter and go to great lengths to see people smile or double over in laughter, because that puts them at ease. Humor has a way of bringing us together; it's comfortable, non-threatening. Somehow it seemed irreverent to summon my sense of humor when I was sure I might be facing death... but if they were going to take my breast I wanted it to be the right one... quite literally... so I wrote the words **TAKE THIS ONE** on a small post-it note and put it on my right breast just before surgery. I understand that now body parts are visibly marked before removal. I'd like to think that maybe I started that movement. This act gave me great pleasure and I considered it a moment of relief, laughing at my written instructions to my surgeon. I got great pleasure out of imagining him laughing too when he pulled back the surgical sheets.

For the particular breast cancer I had, mastectomy was the only treatment. For many women, after surgery they endure months of chemotherapy and radiation. These are the women who battle breast cancer with the best and only weapons that we have: chemotherapy and radiation. They are my heroes.

After a period of recuperation, I returned to work as quickly as I could, wanting to put breast cancer in my past. My first day back I ran into a coworker, "Kate (he always insisted on calling me Kate, despite knowing my name), I haven't seen you in a while. Where have you been?" I was surprised he had not heard about my surgery but I had nothing to hide so I blurted out, "Well I had to have some surgery." "Oh," he said quizzically, "nothing serious I hope." "Well Joe, I had a mastectomy." He looked at me wide eyed, and shot back; "I thought you had those off years ago!" (Okay, so I wasn't known for my chest in those days... and I'm not now either.)

This was a "laughing matters when you have breast cancer" moment. At that instant I realized he didn't care about my breasts, he cared about me... I also realized I was laughing more than I had laughed in weeks and it felt good.

A couple of years passed and I met other women who had had breast cancer. We decided that women diagnosed with breast cancer would benefit from coming together and sharing experiences, not to commiserate about breast cancer but to learn from each other on how to survive with it, to become more educated.

We formed the After Breast Cancer Support Network, wanting women to know that life DOES exist after a breast cancer diagnosis. In 1990 we passed out handmade flyers to the few women we each knew who were breast cancer survivors, inviting them to come together and talk about our collective experiences. In 1990, we only needed a few stamps to send out our handful of meeting notices. Today our mailing list nears one thousand, covering a wide area in Central New York and beyond.

And then, breast cancer is not a laughing matter moment. In our first year, sadly, we lost a member of our group. The breast cancer she had was invasive and difficult to stop; perhaps it was found too late, and perhaps the treatments were not as good twenty-two years ago as they are now.

We were devastated; we didn't know if we could or should go on with our meetings. It was that bold in-your-face reality that women do die from this disease, the disease that had brought us together. But we soon came to realize we needed each other. We needed a forum in which to talk, we needed people to be scared with, friends who would understand our constant worry of cancer returning. And when a woman loses her life to breast cancer we found we need each other even more. We continued our monthly meetings, which have turned into years of meetings... eighteen so far.

In the years that I've been coordinator of this group, I've learned that more than anything humor is a valid medication, no matter where you are in the course of treatment or even when the battle gets rough. Of course it takes a while to see that humor is harmless and needed. Believe me, I did not walk out of my doctor's office doubling over in laughter. It took a while for me to realize that it was okay to laugh, especially if I initiated it. Once I accepted my diagnosis I knew what I had to do to get on with my life. I couldn't see any harm in laughing... if just a little. I also came to realize that there isn't any one of us who can live more than one day at a time anyway, whether you have cancer or not.

Humor is an important defense mechanism; it can help us adjust to the stress of illness and treatment. Being able to laugh can create a sense of power. By helping you adjust to the reality of your illness, it can give you a renewed sense of control over your life. (i.e., a simple way I gained some control by placing the post-it note on my breast).

I've read that scientific studies have found evidence to support a variety of laughter's physical benefits One study found that laughter helps blood vessels function better. Another study shows that laughter causes your brain to release chemicals that relax your muscles and produce pleasure. Still, another study credits laughter with stimulating the body's immune system, which can help fight viruses. And hearty laughter of course stimulates your internal organs.

The ability to laugh is hardwired into our systems and research shows that it's not only good for us, it is contagious. There is a reason sitcoms and stand-up comedy are funnier when we're in a group. When we see someone laugh, our brain seems to activate "mirror neurons" that send us into the same fit of laughter.

It's hard not to feel happy when you're laughing, which explains why laughter and hope go hand in hand. Laughter can provide a sense of perspective on our problems. And it's just plain healthy! The only side effects might be sore sides from laughing hard!

It became apparent that we should devote at least one meeting a year to humor. Not that we don't enjoy humor at all of our meetings. But at our annual humor meeting all the stops are pulled, everything is irreverent. For that hour, laughing matters! For that moment we forget how hard the chemotherapy is, how much the radiation burns skin, how absolutely tired we are with all of it! We simply laugh at the absurd. We are breast cancer survivors... we can laugh at ourselves... we look for the humorous moments that have happened during treatment or with our doctors, we share the laughter, we laugh hard and for that time we feel good.

Just as humor can set the tone for interactions with friends and family members, it can also help establish good communications between people with cancer and their doctors. Being able to share a laugh with your doctor can create a sense of familiarity and trust, which is important for the close relationship that doctors have with their patients. I'm sure my doctor never forgot the post-it note when he started my mastectomy!

Humor works best if the individual can initiate it.

There is a time and a place for wittiness. It would be insensitive to walk up to a newly diagnosed woman and make a joke. But you can help yourself through treatment by devoting some of your time to funny movies, funny books—anything light-hearted. If your friends want to know how they can help you, suggest they visit with a funny DVD and then watch it together.

Most of all, if there is a support group available, become a part of it. Walking into a room and seeing a group of women who have survived breast cancer is the elixir of hope. Their presence is a message that women DO survive this disease. We all need to keep in mind that more women survive breast cancer than not. There is strength in a group that is greater than each of its members.

Yes, life changes after a diagnosis, and for me it was the After Breast Cancer Support Network. This is the most productive and positive element to come out of my breast cancer experience... and perhaps the most significant initiative I've ever done in my life.

Postscript

What can we learn from Karen's story? A lot! Karen was "numb with fear" when first learning of her diagnosis. This is a very normal response to hearing you have breast cancer. But, Karen worked through the fear and grew personally from the experience. She was able to take charge of her fear and her cancer treatment while at the same time maintaining an optimistic attitude. She tells us, "Cancer does have a way of putting things into perspective! Immediately after diagnosis there is a natural tendency to see only the dark clouds, when in fact there really is a blue sky background behind those clouds." The question you might ask is: How did she manage to not only put the breast cancer in perspective, but also be so positive about the experience?

Karen used her sense of humor to deal with the surgery and the cancer. Humor is a great tool because it takes the "sting" out of a threat like breast cancer. When you reduce the threat of cancer, you can put it in its proper perspective.

You can also think about how you might use the experience to help yourself and others, and Karen did this. Breast cancer prompted her to start the After Breast Cancer group. The formation of the ABC group and the friendships that developed are the "gifts" that came from the cancer experience. Karen was able to extract opportunity from the health crisis, turning her cancer into a positive experience. Karen's story has all the ingredients for resilience. Her breast cancer provided post-traumatic growth for Karen. Her ability to organize and develop the ABC group is proof of that growth.

Thank you, Karen.

Two

Mary

I was born in the Mohawk Valley, and I'm the second of five children. I have a brother who is a certified nurse practitioner, one who is a business person, one who is a funeral director, and a sister who works for the Syracuse city schools. I have an undergraduate degree in journalism from Syracuse University. I pursued a law degree at Pace University in New York City. I was a night student and worked during the day. I had some great jobs. I worked in economic development for Queens County and for the city of Yonkers. Now I practice law in Herkimer, New York.

I was diagnosed with breast cancer on May 22, 2002. I had thought that cancerous lumps weren't painful, so when I felt a lump in my right breast that hurt I did not suspect cancer. I saw a doctor immediately just to be sure. So I was very surprised when the doctor told me I had breast cancer and that he wanted to do surgery immediately on the lump that was 1.5 centimeters in size and remove all my lymph nodes. He told me there was lymph node involvement, which is not a good sign.

He was a local doctor, and I just didn't like the look on his face. He looked so scared. I wasn't scared. I found someone else to treat me. I've always been the kind of person who wanted to find out as much as I could about everything, so I read two books about breast cancer in two days. I found out about lymphedema and that removal of all lymph nodes should be avoided if possible. I called people who had had breast cancer to try and get some perspective on what I was facing.

I decided to go to Memorial Sloan Kettering Cancer Center in New York City for treatment. I had my surgery there and was fortunate to have a wonderful surgeon, Dr. Jeanne Petrek, who is now deceased. I settled two cases and had enough money to make the trip—which amounted to almost thirty trips over less than a year. Cancer costs money—there are things that the insurance doesn't pay for like travel and hotels.

After the surgery, I took part in a chemotherapy trial that required treatment every other week for two months and then once a week after that for total chemo treatments twenty-four times. They would hammer us really hard with the heaviest drugs they had, Taxol and Taxotere. I asked my oncologist if she was trying to kill us. I thought my question was funny. She did not laugh.

Out of forty-five women who started the trial, forty-four finished. I did very well, but the scuttlebutt was some women were getting heart failure or heart problems because of the drugs, and in the later part of the trial some of the drugs were discontinued.

My companion for that week and I would take the train to Sloan Kettering on Thursday night and stay until Saturday. I would not feel ill until Sunday night. That was good. Getting sick on an Amtrak train should be avoided. I would always travel with my mom, my sister and niece (who at six years old was used to seeing Aunt Mary without hair), my friends, and sometimes my husband at the time, and my sons. In the winter we would get on the train in Utica, and during better weather we'd drive to Poughkeepsie and take the commuter train to Grand Central Station.

My mother, who is now eighty-one years old, was a great source of support for me. She's a trooper who raised the five kids. At forty-four years of age she was a widow with children ranging from twenty-one to twelve years old. She truly is my hero. I am thankful I got some of that good stuff. She or "the companion of the week" would stay over at the Leo House, which is run by the Sisters of St. Agnes. It's in Manhattan on 23rd Street, and they offer people who are ill a place to stay at really reasonable rates.

I have to say that I think chemotherapy makes you want to shop. I shopped when I was in New York (EVERY time), saw eight Broadway plays, and ate wonderful food, although after awhile the chemo affects your taste buds and you can't really taste anything after a time. I felt sort of like those food columnists who write: "and my companion had *** which was too dry." After a time, I couldn't taste so I asked my companion to taste my food and tell me whether it was good or not.

You change with the treatments. Your body changes. The weirdest thing was no hair in my nose. Sounds crazy but without hair in your nose, your nose bleeds and is very dry. Because of the surgery I lost feeling under my arm. Due to chemotherapy I have limited feeling in my toes and fingertips (neuropathy, which is not uncommon). Chemo does a number on the body. After fifty years of treating people with those toxins, there should be something better. All you researchers: "Help!" But thanks for saving me in the meantime.

One of the things I did to help me through treatment was to focus. I focused on this situation like I had focused on the bar exam because I wanted to get it right the first time. I had radiation treatments, too, for thirty-five days. Unlike the chemo, which took an entire day, radiation treatments didn't last long. Two-and-a-half Hail Marys and it was over. I did say those prayers each time and got great comfort indeed. Getting undressed and dressed was longer than the treatment. The kids today think tattoos are cool—I have them too on my chest. They were used to plot the radiation rays. Radiation was a piece of cake compared to chemo.

I never cried until treatment was all over. I can remember going to my first Relay for Life where people walk all day and night for two days to raise funds for the American Cancer Society. At night, there are hundreds of candles lit all around the running track at the local school. The candles are in bags called luminaries. There are names on the bags for those who died and for those who lived. It took me two years to attend my first relay to get the courage to go. On my first walk around the track, I was reading the bags. I was shocked when I read my name "In honor of Mary I." I cried. I cried while I was walking all around the track after that. It was hard to stop crying. I was moved.

Because of my experiences, I started a local chapter of the ABC (After Breast Cancer Support Network), and for two years we had speakers come: nutritionists, pharmacists, social workers, respiratory therapists, and a massage therapist who came and talked about lymphatic drainage. I am very big on education. Education saves people and helps us with stuff we never imagined. Have those mammograms.

I also take part in a program called Casting for Recovery, and I am now a Participant Coordinator. Every year the Carbone family sponsors a retreat at their lovely home in the Adirondacks where women are taught to fly fish; everything is catered with wonderful food made by two gourmet chefs. On one night, Don Carbone himself cooks—a real pig roast with all the trimmings. They spoil us wonderfully and the women really bond. In between, we learn how to fish.

During the later part of my treatment, I lived with my mother. I needed the help because the cancer treatment weakens the body so. I can recall going from the Lazy Boy to the couch and back again until it was time for bed. I could hardly keep my eyes open. I had no hair or eyebrows and a round face from the steroids. Was I a sight, though I never minded being bald. At the end of the day, I would find my bed would be turned down with my night gown laid out nicely on the bedspread—I teased my mother that all that was lacking was a piece of chocolate on the pillow. She seriously asked me if I really wanted that—she was ready to comply!

At the end of my treatment I only worked a few days a week. It is funny when you have cancer. I lost a lot of business—people think either you are going to die or they don't want to bother you. I am still recovering from my business losses but things will be fine.

Every day is a blessing for me. Having cancer was the best thing that ever happened to me. I wasn't really living, just going through life. I thought I was immortal and there would always be time. I have a better life than I did before. I had the courage to rid myself of a bad marriage but at a great personal loss because I lost my children along the way, too, although things are getting better now.

I am back to practicing law. I try to be mindful about what I do as I am doing it. I do a lot of volunteer work;

I plant and smell my flowers. I exercise and try to eat right. I am happy for the day. I laugh a lot and out loud. I joke. I love my family. I love my friends. I really love my dog. I really amaze myself. Everybody should be as lucky as I am.

Postscript

Mary says breast cancer was "the best thing that happened to me. I wasn't really living, just going through life." Her story is a good example of post-traumatic growth. Mary's life actually improved after having breast cancer. She grew as a person and now is able to appreciate life in a way that is more genuine, more joyful, and certainly more meaningful. How did this transformation take place?

Mary has the take-charge, proactive attitude that characterizes so many resilient breast cancer survivors. She researched the information about breast cancer herself, found the best place to seek treatment, and actively chose the physician she wanted to work with. Mary was an active participant in her own care. She knew what she needed and proceeded to surround herself with people who would foster her sense of hope. She also set little goals for herself and focused on those goals. This helped Mary because focusing on small goals helps a person stick with the treatment plan.

Mary also has a challenge orientation and an optimistic attitude. We see this in a number of ways. First, Mary has a sense of humor. She was able to joke about the more problematic aspects of chemotherapy. Finding the humor in chemotherapy reduced the negativity associated with this uncomfortable situation and therefore made it more manageable.

Mary also extracted the opportunity out of her cancer experience. She made the trips to New York City for the chemotherapy more palatable by using them as an occasion to shop or see a play. In other words, Mary lessened the "sting" of chemotherapy by engaging in pleasurable activities before and after the treatment. This strategy reduced the negativity and threat associated with the chemotherapy.

She also actively found ways to get around its side effects. For example, when she temporarily lost her sense of taste, she had others describe for her what they were eating and used her own imagination to make up for her lack of taste. These strategies helped reduce the temporary losses associated with the side effects of treatment.

Mary had allies in her fight with cancer. Her mother and sister were frequent companions on the trips to New York City. Her mother in particular provided both emotional and instrumental support. Now Mary is providing that support to others. Mary's experience with cancer empowered her to rid herself of a bad relationship. It also helped her "seize the moment" and appreciate each day as a blessing.

Thank you, Mary.

Three

Sheila

I grew up in the metropolitan New York area on Long Island at a time when the area was very rural. I have a younger brother who is still alive who has also had cancer experiences. I went to college. Since I got married we've lived in a number of places up and down the eastern part of the United States. I've now been in Utica for about twenty-three years. I was a math teacher and taught in New York, Massachusetts, Alabama, Pennsylvania, and back to New York. My mother at ninety-two has more energy than I do. It's hard to keep up with her and she's doing fine.

I was diagnosed in the summer of 2002. It was very interesting. Everybody I saw along the way said there's no need to rush, nothing urgent, but everybody was opening doors and things happened very quickly. I had the surgery within a month of the time that I was diagnosed.

The time frame was very short. I went for a routine mammogram. The doctor reading the x-ray said, "There's something here, you'd better go see somebody."

I went for a stereotactic biopsy and they determined that, yes, it was cancer. I had two small cancers. One of the most important things for me was that my gynecologist called me at 10:00 one night and said, “Okay, this is where we are. This is the procedure I’d like you to follow. I’d like you to have these particular x-rays, I’d like you to do this, I’d like you to have this kind of surgery,” and he described the procedures as best he could. Everybody I talked to along the way described the procedures precisely the same way and I found that very comforting.

I had the surgery in Cooperstown at Bassett Hospital and when I met with the surgeon the first time she examined me, she looked at the x-rays, and she sat down and played with her gray ponytail. Then she said, “Okay, what are we going to do about this cancer?” And I looked at her and said, “You’re going to take care of it.”

I’m a very lucky lady. I have a large circle of very caring friends. I don’t have any family nearby. My friends were just superb. Everybody was supportive and meals kept coming. I was very fortunate. I was very comfortable. The surgery was not a difficult experience for me.

I had the surgery on a Monday, and I play in a regular bridge group on Wednesday afternoons, and I felt so well, and I was just bored because there wasn’t very much that I could do. I said to my husband “I have to go because I’ve nothing else to do.” So somebody came and picked me up and I went. We play a lot but we don’t keep score and we may correct each other, which is a wonderful thing. One of the things that surprised me most about this whole experience is that I'm generally a private person about things about myself. Somehow I found it very easy to talk about this and to share my experiences. I was kind of surprised at myself.

I was very positive right through breast cancer. I just knew it was all going to be taken care of. As a matter of fact, we went to an elder hostel shortly after my surgery before I started the radiation, and one of the courses in the elder hostel was about writing your life story. During the course of the week we had several writing assignments, and I remember I was writing that I just considered this a small detour in the road of life. I was a very lucky lady.

I do volunteer, too. I make phone calls and I visit people and I talk to people, and whenever I hear of anybody who is having a problem I send a note and I call or something, because I just think it's so important to know that there are others out there who have been there. When they look at me, and I don't think you would have any indication I've had breast cancer, they can think, oh, she did that, too.

I belong to a gym and we take a Pilates class. The teacher, who is also about my age, had breast cancer during the summer and when she went for radiation the whole class tried to be very supportive. When she finished her radiation we had a luncheon. We had a party; we're very, very supportive of one another.

I'm generally a positive person and fortunately have not had many illnesses. This is not going to get in my way—I'm going! My mother is a fantastic role model. I visited her in February for a week. She's ninety-two and she gave an hour lecture at a biography club and then we went to lunch. I consider her a role model, definitely. And my mother-in-law was a very positive influence and my husband.

I don't know that "healing" is the word I would use to describe what I feel, but I think maybe it's part of my situation. My husband is a clergyman, and I visit people who have a death in the family or where there is illness or sad occasions as well as happy occasions. That is just part of me, so I don't know that I would say it's healing, or that it's a healing experience in particular. I think there is one more thing.

I'm an extremely fortunate person. I was never ill through all of this. I don't think I had any fear at any time. I just had a lot of confidence in what everybody was going to do for me and to me and just went for it. It was just all so matter-of-fact. I think the very fact that my gynecologist had explained so much in such great detail and that everything fell into place precisely as he had indicated was all very comforting. I had great confidence in all my physicians because they agreed with one another about how to proceed. I just knew it was going to work.

Postscript

Sheila's story reflects many of the familiar themes of resilience. She tells us that she is a positive person, and that is certainly evident in the way she thought about her cancer experience: "I just considered this (breast cancer) a small detour in the road of life and I was on my way."

Sheila was confident with her course of treatment and was able to focus on "living" throughout her treatment. She maintained her normal routine as much as she possibly could. She considered herself a "fortunate" person even when she was in the midst of the breast cancer treatment, and this is a critical point. Sheila's optimistic attitude about herself pervaded her own definition of her situation. Having breast cancer did not change her perception of herself and as a result, she was able to put it in the context of her wider life experience. She now volunteers and offers support whenever someone is having a problem. Her experience broadened her life to include helping others who've had breast cancer.

But are there "protective factors" in Sheila's story that may have contributed to her optimistic and giving attitude? The research on resilience points to a number of factors in Sheila's life that may have contributed to her ability to maintain such a positive and optimistic outlook. For one, Sheila has a supportive family. Her husband and wide circle of caring friends provided her with the social support she needed. She had family and friends that she could talk with. And she had friends who provided her with instrumental support like prepared meals.

Sheila's mother was also a role model. No doubt it was her mother's example that taught her how to think positively, how to cope, and how to graciously accept support from others when necessary. Sheila herself was well aware of the value of seeking out positive role models in times of crisis. She says, "I just think it's so important to know others who have been there." She was also experienced in helping others with her husband and his ministry.

These helping experiences provide people the opportunity to earn the support and respect of others. Also, one who has helped others learns what kind of support to provide during different times of need. In Sheila's case, her history helping others may have contributed to her network of social supports and to her ability to use them so well.

Finally, the medical personnel who cared for Sheila contributed significantly to her resilient recovery. Their willingness to spend the time and explain the procedures and course of treatment is a good example of solid informational support. The detailed knowledge Sheila gained helped her maintain her confidence because she knew what to expect. It eliminated the stress and fear that comes from not knowing.

Thank you, Sheila.

Four

Nancy

First I'm going to preface this: over the last five years I decided, whether my grandchildren want it or not, I am going to write down how I lived my life when I was young. I was going to quit this when I married, but somehow when I got to that point I just kept going, so I now have fifty pages of material about my life and my family's life. Included in that is the story of my breast cancer. I wrote it as part of this personal memoir. I'm the glass half-empty instead of the glass half-full. Plus there's a little difference in that I was diagnosed in 1988 and there was a total difference in terms of the amount of information available and in terms of the number of people who had been walking around as breast cancer survivors, or at least the ones we knew about. The whole breast cancer environment was totally different in 1988.

I was born in Utica. I'm an only child. I lived in Utica until I was about eight and my father died. We moved away for just a year but then we came back. We moved to New Hartford when I was ten. My mother taught school there. I graduated from New Hartford High School. I went to Cornell University, got a master's degree in library science from Syracuse, and went back to Ithaca and worked four years at Cornell in the library.

I was married and came to Clinton, lived in Clinton a year, but then we left Clinton. We found a piece of land in New Hartford and built a house, and I worked for two years at Hamilton College library and then had my children. Then I went back. I was a librarian part time at St. Elizabeth's School of Nursing for thirty-two years. So, once I landed there I stayed. I retired in 1997 and still live in New Hartford. I have two boys and a girl. Our son lives in New Hartford, the oldest, and the other two live in Boston. I also have four grandchildren.

As far as I know I'm cancer-free. Breast cancer people can never really say they are cancer-free. Their cancers can return and even though some cancers are considered cured after five years, breast cancer is not. It's unlikely that mine will come back. The first one was diagnosed in 1988; I had a second primary breast cancer in the opposite breast in 1991. So, I've had cancer twice, but it's not a metastasis. It's not a spread of the original cancer; it's two separate cancers.

My absolute first thought was, oh now I know what I'm going to die from. I thought, I don't know when, but I know that now I've been diagnosed with breast cancer that will be my cause of death. But I've totally changed my mind now. I think that that was the time. You didn't talk about cancer, and there were several people who came up to me because I talked about my illness. There were also several people who came up to me and told me that they had breast cancer, and I had no idea that they had it.

But the other reason that it struck me particularly hard was that when I had the biopsy, which was a surgical biopsy, and I was still there in the hospital for that, the initial pathology results came back negative. So I went home; it was November, and I remember watching a movie or television that night and just feeling so wonderful and thinking, oh, now I can get on with my Christmas shopping and everything to do with the holiday.

The next day the doctor called and said, "We're very sorry, but we made a mistake, and will you please call your husband and come to the office as soon as possible?" So we did and he explained that this was a minimal cancer. Nowadays, I would have a lumpectomy and I would be watched carefully and have radiation. At that point they did a mastectomy, and the doctor also told us, including my husband who was panicked, that it didn't look good. He expected that it would spread and he told me that the most common areas for spread were lungs, liver, brain, and bone. And that wasn't really what I wanted to hear on that day. So my experience with that particular episode was not good.

My husband didn't tell me this, but he met my

doctor in the post office and my doctor said that he wished women would not talk about their breast cancers among themselves because they don't understand very much and they think that because "Mrs. A." had one treatment then that's what they should have and that they don't understand that all breast cancers are different. He said everyone's case is very individual, so they really should just keep their mouths shut and listen to the doctor.

I feel completely different about cancer because I have survived for sixteen years, and there is nothing that will change your mind like survival. I also feel very differently because I had an understanding of this whole process once I went through the first surgery and because it was so minimal that I did not need chemotherapy.

A good acquaintance of mine was one of the founders of the ABC group, and I started going to the ABC meetings, which I still attend. And over the years I have learned and read a tremendous amount. I joined Reach to Recovery, and I've talked to many, many women and others that I just happen to know: friends, cousins, you know, all sorts of people who have had breast cancer. I try to stay as informed as I can so that I can help people.

The whole scene is so different and so much more positive now, and so many more women are getting mammograms that the proportion of early cancers detected has risen tremendously. So, for all those reasons, new drugs and a lot of things, it's more positive now.

Support is important; the ABC Group was started very soon after my cancer, probably about 1989, and it was Karen Christensen who is still with it and a woman by the name of Theresa Flihan who was my friend and Bobbi somebody who moved out of the area after about two years. It meets at Faxton about once a month. We have wonderful speakers who talk about everything. Dr. Joseph fulfills two purposes with the group. She provides us with extremely interesting information and she also tells us very humorous stories. Humor is a big part of this whole thing in terms of recovery so she does more than her share.

As far as treatment is concerned, my daughter-in-law took Adriamycin and Taxol and something else, but she had to have her heart checked. Now the first bunch I was on was FAC; I don't even know what the letters stand for. It made our resistance so low that we had to self inject with Neupogen because that raises your white blood count. Chris would put it in the needle for me and I would inject myself. This was during the treatment to raise the white blood cells and prevent anemia. When you're in it you just do what you've got to do.

Though the prognosis may be excellent, a cancer diagnosis can be a defining moment in one's existence. Psychologically, life is forever divided into "before cancer" and "after cancer." For me it meant developing a keener empathy for others similarly afflicted. Besides joining a support group, I trained to be a Reach to Recovery volunteer. Periodically I spoke with, and tried to encourage, other breast cancer victims, either during their hospital stays or at home. Through ABC, I participated in several panel discussion programs, modeled for fashion show fundraisers, and even told my story in a video made for recently diagnosed cancer clients. On the personal side, I learned to better appreciate the simple pleasures of daily living.

My annual mammograms for the opposite breast were clear until August 1991, when a small suspicious lump appeared on the extreme left edge. When the biopsy revealed cancer, there was no doubt that a second mastectomy must be done. A wave of depression and an, "I can't go through all that again," mood set in. Trying to divert my mind, we made one last camping trip before heading for the hospital in late August.

Again my lymph nodes were clean, but the tumor itself, about 1.2 cm, was more aggressive than some. Since my estrogen receptors were also negative, I was prescribed six months of adjuvant chemotherapy. I took daily pills and once a week for two weeks an intravenous injection of two drugs. The second two weeks of each month I went without treatment. Six months of this left me fatigued, nauseous, and without most of my hair, including eyebrows. I did, however, manage to show up for my part-time library job and to continue with an almost normal schedule of outside activities.

Mercifully, by March 1992, the treatments were over. My body gradually returned to normal, although my hair never regained its original bounce, and my eyebrows only partially grew back. Periodic checkups and tumor marker blood tests led to some scary moments, but no return of the cancer. As the years passed I became more confident that the odds were on my side.

I would say to the newly diagnosed do as much research as you can and just keep real positive because you'll get through it. There is a time when your treatment will be over and you'll educate yourself. Don't always rely on just what the doctor says. If you want, get a second opinion. You have to take responsibility and I think the best thing that I did was not going to that surgeon.

Postscript

Nancy's personal story is compelling because she was able to grow despite her initial negative experience with breast cancer. In her case, the first surgeon she consulted painted the most negative prognosis despite his contention that the cancer was "minimal." Nancy took charge and sought out a different surgeon. This is a good example of the proactive take-charge attitude we see with resilience and post-traumatic growth.

She also joined other women in Reach to Recovery and became involved in the newly formed ABC group. She learned to evaluate information about breast cancer critically, and she used strategies such as humor to maintain her focus and proactive attitude. Nancy grew from the experience of breast cancer. She tells us, "I felt self-empowered... a cancer diagnosis can be a defining moment in one's existence...for me it meant developing a keener empathy for others similarly afflicted."

Nancy's treatment was at a time when breast cancer was perceived as a "death sentence." It was also a time when the surgical treatment for breast cancer routinely involved a mastectomy. Her doctor's expressed opinion that woman should not talk with each other but rather listen to "the doctor only" reflects the old time notion that health and illness are experienced in a social vacuum. Now we know better, and doctors often refer newly diagnosed women to support groups.

It is true that each person's case is different from the next. It is also true that accurate information about cancer and treatment, along with appropriate social supports, contributes significantly to positive outcomes for breast cancer. Nancy's story certainly illustrates the power of support and the need to assume responsibility for one's own care.

Thank you, Nancy.

Five

Anonymous

I am thirty years old, a mother of three young children: two, four, and ten. I have been married eleven years to my high school sweetheart. I was born and raised in the Mohawk Valley on a farm, went to the local school, and still have friends that I have known for twenty-six years. I am a middle child and both my parents are still alive and work on the farm.

I work as a grade school teacher and have been for about five years in the same district. I live with my husband and children in a home in the country. We recently built it in the same school district we both attended. We want our children to have the same opportunities we had in a small school.

I was diagnosed in May of 2005. I went to the doctor because my husband felt a lump in my left breast. I wasn't really concerned with this because I was young and healthy and had no family history of cancer. I remember the doctor telling me he would like to do a biopsy as soon as possible, and I also was scheduled for a mammogram.

At that time I finally got nervous. Although I am an educated person, I tried to deny the fact that this could be serious. I had my mammogram the next morning and remember the doctor telling me it was highly suspicious. My biopsy was done the next day by a local surgeon who came recommended by a woman I trusted. At this point I was scared.

After it was confirmed that I had cancer, I had to be strong and tell those closest to me. I am a private person so I kept it relatively secret. Not many people were told. I did cry in private, but put on an optimistic front in public. My husband and my best friend were the most helpful. I kept my kids during the hospital stays. I had two lumpectomies and opted for a mastectomy after I couldn't get clear margins. This was a final decision, and no chemo or radiation was needed, so I could resume my life sooner.

Something positive came out of this. I am a stronger person who takes every day for what it is. I don't wish away my life. My challenges are few. I do have to watch what I carry because I am still healing. I don't hesitate to ask for help.

Advice I would give would be to always check for abnormalities. You are not free from the disease. Anyone can have cancer and for those lucky enough to avoid the disease, help those less fortunate.

Postscript

Anonymous' story begins with the normal feeling many experience when first given the diagnosis of breast cancer...fear. However, Anonymous does not allow the fear to consume her. Rather, she proceeds with the treatment and deals with the stress of the early diagnosis in her own personal way.

Anonymous' style is different from the other women described in this book. She found solace by crying in private, but then "put on an optimistic front in public." Her ability to cry in private and then present an optimistic public persona is an indication of Anonymous' ability to take charge of her own feelings. Her need to deal with the cancer in a private way is perfectly appropriate and is an example of the differences in each individual's coping style.

Despite her private style of coping, Anonymous still had her husband and best friend to turn to. The value of social support applies regardless of one's own personal coping style. Anonymous relied on her friend and husband for emotional and instrumental support. They recognized her need for privacy and personal time and were available when she needed someone to listen. She grew from the experience. She tells us, "I am a stronger person who takes every day for what it is. I don't wish away my life."

Thank you, Anonymous.

Six

Pat

My name is Pat. I am seventy-three years old and a widow of four years. I was born in Little Falls Hospital and was raised in the town of Newport until my late teen years when my family moved to the neighboring town of Poland. I am the younger of two children; I have an older brother. I graduated from high school and attended one year of business school at CCBI in Syracuse, New York. I then became a secretary for approximately five years, a cafeteria aide for three years, a reading aide for four years, and worked in a dress shop for approximately two years before I became a housewife, raising three children of my own with my husband. My grandmother had breast cancer in which she had a bilateral mastectomy and eventually died from complications.

I was diagnosed in early September 1996. I underwent what the doctor called a left partial masectomy, I called it a lumpectomy, on September 10, 1996. The cancer was found by a routine mammogram that I received yearly due to my family history.

There was no evidence of a palpable lump and no signs or symptoms of cancer.

I was told about my cancer over the telephone in a very matter of fact way by the physician after the biopsy was done. I was shocked at the news, but my husband was there to comfort me at the time of the phone call. I dealt with my cancer by keeping busy and deciding I was going to fight and not let this destroy my life. I kept busy with all the tests and appointments. I am a very strong woman. I had lost a son to suicide just two years prior to the diagnosis. Cancer was nothing compared to that, and if I could manage to get through that this disease was not going to stop me.

When I was asked if anyone was particularly helpful, I do not recall any one person standing out. As I said the doctor was not helpful at all and just treated me very casually. Nothing great about any nurses either. I was very upset that no one told me about arm exercises after surgery. It was many months later when I found these out from a friend in conversation. My husband and family were very supportive, although when you ask my children about it, they state they know little about the whole ordeal.

I was in the hospital just overnight and the only obstacle was the drain. I frequently mentioned how I hated the drain. I only experienced pain with the drain and received only Tylenol for that. I was upset about little to no information about the recovery period in general. I received radiation therapy five days a week from October 10 to November 25. There were a total of thirty-three treatments. During my radiation period my husband was diagnosed with prostate cancer, and he underwent surgery a few days after my last radiation treatment.

On a positive note, I value life more and encourage my daughter to receive routine mammograms and my son prostate exams. The only challenges I have encountered have been the routine mammograms and uncertainty of the cancer reappearing. My only advice to others is to stay positive, keep going on through life even if you do not want to, and do everything they tell you to do. Make sure you receive and understand all the information, and do not be afraid to ask questions. And keep busy and work as long as you can. When asked what past experiences helped me through my own experience, I stated that I have become a strong individual from previous life-altering experiences (my youngest son's death). Keep a positive attitude.

Postscript

Pat is no stranger to adversity. Prior to her diagnosis of breast cancer, she had dealt with the death of her son. Her proactive attitude and behavior are evident right from the time of diagnosis, when she says, "I dealt with my cancer by keeping busy and deciding I was going to fight and not let this destroy my life." Pat engaged in routine activity to maintain her sense of control and fighting spirit. She, like many other women in this book, accepted the social support of family and friends. The experience of having breast cancer, along with the other traumas Pat endured, made her more keenly aware of the value of life.

Unfortunately for Pat, medical personnel did not appear to be supportive. The health care system, with the "matter of fact" attitude of the treating physician and the poor education she received about the procedures and aftercare, in many ways created more distress for Pat. This was unfortunate, especially given Pat's personal history of loss. However, with the support of her husband and family, Pat overcame the obstacles. She adjusted and grew despite her negative experience with the health care system. Her story speaks to the resilience of the individual and the power of the support of family and friends.

Thank you, Pat.

Seven

J.L.P.

I was born in Rome, New York, but grew up in Westmoreland, New York. I was the only daughter and the middle child. I graduated from Westmoreland Central High School and was a two-year college graduate of Mohawk Valley Community College in accounting and have a college diploma in secretarial. I am married and live at home with my spouse. I had the initial surgery in November of 2002, and in January of 2003 had follow-up surgery.

I was not prepared for the diagnosis and went alone thinking the result would be benign. I was shocked and found it hard to keep my emotions together, almost in disbelief. In order to deal with the diagnosis I talked to loved ones. I spent sessions with family and my doctor to discuss the treatment options and pros and cons of each. My doctor answered all questions over several hours.

My son helped by researching treatment options and shared info. My daughter helped by researching cancer types, treatment options, stats, and shared information.

My husband helped during the recovery period, and my granddaughter assisted with the nursing care.

I had decreased mobility of my arm with associated pain, so I did physical therapy activities religiously. Bathing was a problem, so I bought bath pillows to help me sit up. I also purchased wigs in advance in case I lost my hair, which helped with positive attitude.

Some of my close friends withdrew and did not support me during the surgery and recovery process, and then others that I felt were casual friends became very supportive and helpful during that process. Some people have the attitude that once the surgery is done, the person is fully recovered; life goes on unchanged, as it was before it ever happened. I learned to appreciate each day and recognize the good things that come along with it. I have special feelings for other women with breast cancer and can be a support and resource to them.

Surgery and recovery are major challenges. The biopsy was a painful procedure, more than anticipated. The emotional challenge is not to dwell on cancer and project its return in the future and to remain positive. Radiation was frightening, mentally challenging, physically challenging because you don't entirely know about what the radiation does to the body, and the burns from the radiation make it difficult to wear typical clothing.

Having a major surgery earlier that could've had an adverse impact on my life and having very positive results from it taught me to not give up and not lose hope for the future. I wish someone had told me ahead of time that I wouldn't be able to wear a bra following surgery, so I could've shopped ahead of time for an accommodating wardrobe. I also started having a really hard time with the pain of radiation burns and swelling that followed. I had swelling for a year and a half after radiation therapy and hadn't realized that would or could happen. I had to get a different car because my car was a standard, and it became too painful to drive with the affected arm that they removed the lymph nodes from. One of the medications I was on following my surgery needed to be changed later because it made me lose inches of my hair. I relied more on friends for support, rather than on family, because I felt my family was already emotionally burdened with the situation.

It's important not to listen to details about other people's breast cancer if they are giving negative details. Research and learn as much as you can about your diagnosis. Keep a positive mind frame. Make sure you get your mammograms because that's what allowed mine to be caught early. If you know someone with breast cancer offer to be there if needed, open to talk, send a message or card "think-of-you" gestures. Don't say nothing at all, and don't be "pushy"!

Postscript

J.L.P.'s response to her diagnosis is both normal and familiar: "I was shocked and found it hard to keep my emotions together." J.L.P. did adapt with the help of her family and friends. J.L.P.'s family pitched in, and each one of them gathered important information for her. This information enabled her to make a decision, which is the proactive, take-charge behavior so important to breast cancer patients.

They were also there to comfort her by listening to her concerns and fears. Sometimes, just expressing negative feelings helps to relieve them, and having family members willing to listen is so helpful. J.L.P.'s doctor was also supportive. In her case, the doctor provided the informational support she needed to understand her options. The doctor did not make the decision for J.L.P.; rather, he helped her to make an educated decision for herself.

J.L.P. also took charge of her situation. She knew that she needed to maintain a positive attitude. When losing her hair represented a potential threat to her optimism, J.L.P. purchased a wig before her treatment began. This is a great example of the kind of problem solving that comes from a proactive attitude.

J.L.P. also learned valuable lessons about friends and friendship. Sometimes it takes a "crisis" like breast cancer to know who your real friends are. Some of J.L.P.'s close friends withdrew. This was a major disappointment and contributed to the stress already created by the diagnosis of breast cancer. However, having so called "casual" friends come forth and be supportive was reassuring and revealing. Ultimately, the breast cancer provided the opportunity to know true friendship and appreciate each day for its uniqueness. This is the gift that J.L.P. derived from breast cancer.

Thank you, J.L.P.

Eight

Lealo

I was born in Brooklyn. I have four sisters and five brothers and we were a totally dysfunctional family. I didn't live with my parents. I moved from one place to the other. I came from a dysfunctional family where people molested people and things like that, so I had very poor self-esteem for a while until I grew up and taught myself better. I'm African-American and I have mental illness, schizophrenia and bipolar disorder, and that is one of the things that I had to deal with when I found out that I had breast cancer.

I was diagnosed with breast cancer in November 2000. I had a biopsy on the sixteenth, and on the seventeenth my doctor called me and said that I had breast cancer. Well, she didn't say it so bluntly, but she said, "You have breast cancer," and she said it was noninvasive. When she said it, I didn't hear all the rest. All I heard was, "You've got breast cancer." She scheduled an appointment for me to see Dr. Tyler in Syracuse on Monday, and this was on Friday.

So I didn't have an inkling of how I was going to

get there because I had a vehicle, but my vehicle didn't go very far. You know, I just used it to go shopping and such. I called one friend of mine and she took me there, I drove, and we made it there and back. I was scheduled for my surgery for December 4, and, since I'm on SSI, I have Medicaid. But since I have a vehicle, Medicaid said they couldn't transport me to Syracuse. That was a bad situation all around.

The first thing that I would like to say about being diagnosed with breast cancer is that first you get shocked, and then after a while you talk to people who are survivors and find out there's hope. So that's the important thing: to talk about your breast cancer issues with a survivor. The survivors will give you details that no doctor or no book can really tell you because they are people that you're personally talking to, not reading about. You can ask them questions and they can answer your questions. I had such an experience. I went to Mental Health Connections and the director herself had had breast cancer, and she's a five-year survivor. So my therapist got me to talk to her because I was highly upset.

She told me, "You know a five-year survivor. I had chemotherapy and I had radiation. Radiation is the worst. You have to listen to what the doctor tells you, and do what the doctor tells you, and everything will be alright." So I took that idea and I ran with it. You know, I said, "Okay there's hope," and I said, "Breast cancer is not the end." Okay, I got this from a five-year survivor. I can do this, you know, I can do this breast cancer thing.

To get back to the part about getting to Syracuse for my surgery, I work at Human Technologies Corporation and they are the most wonderful people to work for because they are a corporation committed to the excellence of people working with disabilities and barriers to employment. I told my supervisor about the cancer when I got off the phone with my doctor. She gave me a big hug. Then there's another supervisor; she gave me a big hug, and in the meantime they found out I didn't have a way to Syracuse. One of my supervisors said, "Well, if you can't find a way I'll give you the money."

But there was another lady, Bridget, who was a benefit specialist. I went to her and she said, "Look, I'm not supposed to give you this telephone number but I'm going to give you the telephone number for the commissioner of Medicaid transportation, and you talk to her and tell her your situation." I spoke to the lady and she said, "Okay, you talk to the supervisor and tell her to speak to me," and they hooked it up. I got to Syracuse. The morning of my surgery I went to Syracuse by myself, but the two supervisors that I spoke of called me.

They also came over after I got there and were there before I went into surgery and they stayed with me until I went into surgery. They waited and they were there when I woke up from surgery. Now that was the greatest thing. I have a daughter who had lived in the area, but she had moved to Brooklyn for a while and I was up there by myself. I have a son but he was in Korea in the Army. My other son lives in Long Island, but he works and has a family to take care of, so he just couldn't pop up right away. My other daughter lives in Jersey and didn't have the means to come here. So, I was in the hospital and they told me, "Well, you're going home tomorrow," but I still had this drain to drain the fluids out. I said "I can't go home with this drain. I don't know what to do with this; I can't go."

When I first got breast cancer, the next person that I talked to after Kathy Hurtz was Kathy Peters. I had just done Making Strides in October and there I was diagnosed in November, so all I needed to do was to call the American Cancer Society Patient and Family Services. She told me, "Okay, I'll come up to see you in the hospital," and she did. She came up to see me in the hospital, and I told her about my situation and not wanting to go home with the drain. She said, "Well don't worry; I'll get you a visiting nurse. You just go home and you'll be alright." Then my son called me and said, "Mom, I'm on my way up there." So that was wonderful, too.

My son came all the way from Long Island in the bad weather. He took me home and he was there with me fixing breakfast and he took care of me. I was moving around too much and my drain started to leak. I panicked and thought oh my God, I pulled it out, but it had just loosened up enough for the fluids to come down the side of the tube. He went to the store and bought me gauze and stuff and bandaged me up. That felt good, all of it.

I have this to say: If you're diagnosed with breast cancer do not keep it to yourself. It's not taboo. It's something that a lot of people get, and you can work with it even if you have to have chemotherapy and all that. You don't have to worry too much because even now they have drugs that they can give you while you're taking chemotherapy so it doesn't make you so sick. Okay, you lose your hair. There's a lady who works for Faxton Breast Cancer Center and they have wigs and all kinds of things you can wear, and they fix you up. They make you look like you're really, really cool. So you don't have to worry about losing your hair. Once again I say don't keep it to yourself. Tell somebody cause there's a wealth of information out there. You can call the American Cancer Society at 1-800-ACS-2345, and you can get information about any kind of cancer, and if they don't have the information right at hand they'll find it for you and they will direct you to things.

To sum it up, I got more involved. I got to speak for the Relay for Life, which is another American Cancer Society function that celebrates and honors the survivors of all cancers and commemorates the people who have passed on. They had a wonderful luminary ceremony. The luminary ceremony is where you take a little white bag, and it says either "in memory of," or "in honor of," and you write the name on it. You can decorate it with the name and at night, around ten o'clock, you light up all the bags all around the track that you walk. It is the most beautiful and moving thing that you could ever see. All the survivors and people, caregivers of survivors, walk around the track. We have our little candles, and it's the most wonderful ceremony. They play the bagpipes and the bagpipes lead the walk. I went on with that and it's just one thing after another. I want to be involved.

My main thing is I got diagnosed at an early stage, stage one, and that's because I had mammograms continuously. It was caught real early, it was noninvasive, and that means that the cancer didn't spread. In the center of the cancer I had a mass, I didn't have a lump. I had what they called a calcification and it's not a lump. That's why I couldn't tell if I had it or not. The mammogram is the only thing that diagnosed me. So in the center of this mass was a part that was invasive. That means it could have spread. They got the whole thing out, and I was blessed not to have invasive cancer, so I didn't have chemotherapy or radiation. I thank my higher power for that, and I'll just say that you get closer to something greater than yourself.

I'm not going to call it God because some people don't believe in God, but there is something greater than yourself. You get closer to this and you feel pretty good.

You feel good inside. I had colon cancer, too. That happened in January of the same year, 2006. That cancer was also caught early. I had a colon resection with no chemotherapy or radiation because it was caught early.

It didn't bother me too much because there was a history of colon cancer in our family, but with the breast cancer I was devastated. I was truly devastated. I didn't know what to think. I felt like somebody had told me I was gonna die. You know, with breast cancer you're gonna die. Like okay, get things together because you're gonna die. But I found out that's not true.

When you get diagnosed with breast cancer there's life; there's a lot of life. There are people who've been survivors for fourteen, twenty-five, thirty years. I've been surviving less than a year. Next month is November and I'll be one-year survivor. And I make fun out of it. I've had a ball. I just really had a ball.

I talk to people and I tell them to get tested, and I found out that men get breast cancer now. That's something that men don't want to hear. They don't have milk ducts and all that stuff, but they have enough breast tissue that they can get breast cancer. Men don't get tested for breast cancer, and that's not a good thing. I've heard of fatalities from men having breast cancer, but they do also survive.

I would have to say I've associated with friends and family, and those are the things, friends, family, and my higher power that are very important to me. The American Cancer Society has been my life, from the Relay for Life right on down to Making Strides Against Breast Cancer. They have a lot of things going on. I can't name them all, but they do education and they have services, and I know they have the Sister Study and another thing called Man to Man. Get in touch with the American Cancer Society. You get cancer, call them.

Postscript

Lealo's story is compelling. Not only did she have to deal with breast cancer, but that same year doctors diagnosed her with colon cancer. Limited material resources, mainly the absence of a reliable car, further complicated her situation, which in turn resulted in difficulty accessing the care she needed. However, Lealo's situation did not immobilize her; she became proactive almost immediately.

She sought out the assistance of her supervisor at work. She got information about breast cancer from other survivors, who then became role models. They were able to kindle the optimistic outlook she expresses when she says, "while you talk to people who are survivors you find out there is hope." She elicited and accepted support from coworkers, from the Cancer Society, and from the Breast Care Center.

Social support and her religious faith made up for what Lealo did not have in terms of material resources.

Her supervisor drove her to Syracuse and stayed with her through the surgery. Then her son came home when he could to help her out, and her deep spiritual belief enabled her to make sense of the cancer experience and realize that she was not alone. All these factors helped Lealo with what appeared to be an overwhelming set of circumstances.

Like other stories in this book, Lealo's reinforces the value of social support. She received emotional and instrumental support from a broad range of people and organizations. No doubt, her early childhood adversity and her own personal struggles with mental illness helped her develop the mental muscle she needed to face these physical problems.

Lealo learned early in life the value of believing and trusting in "something greater than (you)." Her words "the people at my job are like family" and "The American Cancer Society has been my life. From the Relay for Life right on down to Making Strides Against Breast Cancer—that is what I do" show that she developed a new sense of kinship with her coworkers and a renewed sense of purpose.

Thank you, Lealo.

Nine

Yong "Star"

My name is Yong Taylor. I'm from South Korea. I was born in and raised in South Korea. My father worked for a big soap company. My grandfather was a big farmer. I had a brother and sister, but my brother died in the Korean War. My sister died when she was twenty-seven. I'm the youngest one. My mother passed away when I was born, three days later. My father passed away when I was fifteen.

Then I was doing a lot of different things. I was wild because I was rebelling because at a young age I had lost everything I loved. But the one thing saved me was God. My uncle told me, "You speak English." I went to high school in Korea. Then I went to college in Korea. I met my husband right there in a store helping my uncle. When he come over he told me, "Hey you, you're gonna be my wife." I said, "Get out of here." He said, "No, you gonna be my future wife." That's how I met my husband. In 1962 I came here to the United States and we've been married ever since.

My husband was an Olympian. He got the gold

medal. When he came back, he was doing extra duty in California, training soldiers. In 1968 or something like that, he went, but he didn't come home. The company commander called me to tell me he'd had an accident. He was supposed to go to Germany for the Olympics. Well, he couldn't go. Then he was disabled.

I took care of those soldiers coming from the Vietnam War. I had to because my husband was one of them. But they gave me strength. After we came to Utica we used to take care of a lot of Vietnam Eurasians. My house was open twenty-four hours a day, and I was cooking twenty-four hours a day. At that time we had fifty mother-and-children families who came and ate at my house.

In 1995 my husband had a stroke. In 2003 at the end of the year I couldn't take care of him. Then he had another stroke, so he had to go back to Syracuse to the VA hospital. And I was going every single day to take of him. In 2004, I went for a checkup of my breasts. Then they said it was okay, but the doctor did it wrong. People say I should have sued but I don't believe in that. But he did it wrong, so I needed to check up with a regular doctor who I trusted. That's the main thing, "trust." I did not trust that first doctor. He looked at me and said, "Oh, you're here." He never even touched me, just looked at it. I said it hurts, it hurts, but he said, "No, you feeling good."

The doctor said, "Okay, Ms. Taylor, I am going to

send you to a specialist." So they sent me to Oneida and the doctor there did a mammogram and everything. Then he said, "Well I can't tell anything. I have to do a biopsy." So I had another biopsy. Then I told him it hurts here. He said, "Well, we'll see after the biopsy." Two weeks later I went there and the doctor said, "I am going to tell you the truth. You have cancer." I said, "Oh my God, what am I gonna do? I cannot be dying, I got to take care of my husband. Oh God help me, hold my hand God, hold my hand." The doctor said, "Ms. Taylor, I'm going to leave you alone for a minute."

I had a 99 percent chance of recovery with a total mastectomy, and a 35 percent chance with a partial mastectomy. I had a total mastectomy. I did not tell my husband. He had his own problems to deal with. A year and a month later he died. My husband was a very strong believer in God. His whole family was too, but especially my husband. He's gone to God now. His body was cremated. I took him to Miami to the ocean.

My mother-in-law had passed away before my husband. My father-in-law passed away before my husband, but when I came up to Utica he was the most loving, kind person. He was *very* kind. My mother-in-law's mother loved me to death. I have a special friend. Her name is Mabel Johnson. She has been my sister since I came up to Utica. She is my husband's first cousin. Right now she's in New York City. She used to drive a bus then she just had a stroke last year.

God is the first one I look to for support, but besides that it's the people: Little ones, big ones, older ones, it doesn't matter. You reach out. Then they reach out for you. We have good ones and bad ones, but so far all the ones I've met have been good.

Postscript

What does Star's story have to offer someone facing breast cancer? The first and perhaps foremost lesson is Star's faith in God. It helped her deal with adversity throughout her life, starting with the death of her parents and siblings at a young age. It was her faith that helped her through each crisis, including her ordeal with breast cancer. Star also realized the benefits derived from helping others—especially when you yourself are hurting.

After her husband's injury in the service, they opened their home to other veterans of the Vietnam War. She feels that her compassion gave her strength, saying, "I took care of those soldiers coming from the Vietnam War. I had to because my husband was one of them. But they gave me strength." From then on, Star dedicated herself to service, and from this service, she developed a strong sense of purpose and utility.

She also has a rather optimistic view of others: "We have good ones (people) and bad ones, but so far all the ones I've met have been good." She ends her story with some very important advice, "God is the first one I look to for support, but besides that it's people: Little ones, big ones, older ones, it doesn't matter. You reach out. Then they reach out to you."

Thank you, Star.

Ten

Jane

I was born in New York City, in lower Manhattan and did all my education there. I went to the School of Performing Arts where I studied dance. I was really the only one in my modern dance class who went on to college, and I went to the State University of New York at Brockport. There I had the experience of teaching the football team a ballet class, and it was so successful, and I loved it so much, and they had such a great time. I learned so much that I decided that teaching was where my heart was. So I went and got my master's degree in education with a specialty in dance from the University of Michigan, and I'm a teaching artist now. I'm also on the faculty at Colgate University teaching dance.

I was diagnosed in December 1999. Oddly enough, I've always had yearly mammograms and was always fine. My daughter and I decided to go on Weight Watchers; she was almost sixteen then, and we lost thirty pounds each. With that weight loss I started noticing things that I hadn't noticed before, and that's when I discovered my lump, and again I had just had a mammogram that showed nothing. I went to my doctor, who is a friend of mine, and he immediately sent me for another mammogram, which showed nothing, but at the same time he prescribed a sonogram. You can't have a sonogram unless you have a lump. You have to have something for them to sonogram. So when I had the sonogram, there was an interfaced tumor; it's not a perfectly round sphere, but it has prongs on it. There it was.

Then I was sent to the Breast Care Center in Syracuse, because my physician was in Hamilton. I went for a core biopsy, where they take a bit of the tumor and send it to a pathologist. I didn't think anything was wrong, or I was in complete denial; you know, I felt great. I had just lost thirty pounds, I was having a great time, and I had a son in college who was excelling and everything was going great. My husband said that he was coming with me for the report, and I said, "It's really not necessary." I was going to meet a girlfriend for lunch, and he didn't want to take that much time off from work, and I said, "Then don't come. This is nothing, you know, this is really nothing."

It was sad... the surgeon cried with me. I couldn't believe it when she said it was malignant; it was like I was up here, and all of a sudden I was a downer! It was terrible; it was devastating. My mother had breast cancer, but because of her age, she didn't have any treatments. I was young; I was forty-eight, and that's young. I had to drive all the way home from Syracuse to Deansboro, and it was hard.

In retrospect, I wish my husband had come with me. Then all of a sudden I was given all this choice—whether to have a lumpectomy or a mastectomy—and the doctor didn't think it was necessary to have the mastectomy because I wear leotards and tights when I dance, and my body image is important to me. That's the way I was brought up also, with body image. So, I cried. I'm a cry baby.

I was diagnosed with stage one breast cancer, and the recommendation was a lumpectomy and six months of chemo and six weeks of radiation. My son wasn't home at the time, but my husband was a great support. My daughter, who had just turned sixteen, didn't know how to handle all this stuff. That was challenging, and it was on her sixteenth birthday that I told her. It was terrible, but friends really came to the plate. You know, I have dear friends who would bring me food every chemo treatment. Great food: but I couldn't eat anything because after chemo there is such a horrible metallic taste in your mouth. And I gained all my thirty pounds back. But, it was a process.

My husband and I would go to chemo with a positive topic to discuss, and that was very interesting, being in a treatment room where people were literally dying around you as you sit in a chair. There must have been about ten chairs, and you get to meet other people. Everybody's there with a partner of some sort, and, they're just out of it. They're out of it! And we chose that we weren't going to take that approach. I wasn't going to dwell on this thing that was going to kill me, you know, and so that was the attitude.

When I'd been asked, I was put on the borderline for chemo, and my doctor said, "If you want to see your grandchildren, I'd highly recommend this." Since there was no choice for me, as far as I was concerned, we took a real positive approach to it. I taught dance throughout my six months. I only missed two days. And, as I said, my friends brought me food.

I remember very distinctly my forty-eighth birthday. I was chilly and listening to my sixteen-year-old playing the piano. I was lying down and all of a sudden she got up and went into the kitchen and came back giggling and I knew something was up. So I followed her, went back into the kitchen, and there were eight of my girlfriends tossing netting, all different colors of netting, all over the place. You know, it was like life... and it was exuberant, and it was just absolutely gorgeous! And I was thinking to myself, oh my God! Here I had hardly any hair on my head, I felt like shit. This was in March and I'd started chemo in January, so I was just like drained of energy, and I thought so this is, these are eight crazy friends, who really brought me through. My husband was in on it... it was great... it was just great! So that was a high for me.

I'm a Reach To Recovery volunteer now. And I really firmly believe you've got to have a support system. I tell them call me any time of the day, I meet with them when they are newly diagnosed, and we get through this together. I'm still friends with some of the people that I've coached. There were actually some positive things that came from chemo, like my hair. I always had very short hair; it was just always very short all the way around. When you start growing your hair from chemo, it is very curly and kinky, and my hairdresser said, "We're going to keep it." There are other positive things. I think I'm definitely more patient with people who are ill. I listen more than I did before.

I gained back the thirty pounds that I had lost, and you know I attribute losing those thirty pounds to finding my cancer. I've gotten much closer to my children because they lived through it with me but that's not really a challenge, that's a reward.

Sometimes I'm tired, really tired. All that just wrings you right out. This is my fifth year; I'm almost at the end of my fifth year after surgery and I still fall asleep at seven or eight o'clock at night and wake up at 5 a.m. But, I'm tired. So that's my challenge: to persevere and get through the day. I keep on saying this is going to be my last year teaching. How much more can I put this body through in terms of dancing? I come from the school of thought that if you're going to teach dance you've got to dance; you know you just can't sit. I am planning on continuing work. I keep on saying one more year, and I'm going to do one more year again.

I meet a lot of different people through Reach to Recovery. It's when someone newly diagnosed with breast cancer can call a peer volunteer if they want more information. If they want to speak to someone who's had breast cancer, my name is recommended, and I get contacted through the American Cancer Society.

I go into the hospital and I speak about anything that they want to ask me, including my own experience. They're not allowed to mention doctors' names at all. It really depends on where they're at in their stage, if they're in Stage I versus Stage IV. I tell them I went through it. I went through the process. Am I a stronger person for it? I don't know. I'm a more aware person. I'm a more educated person. I'm totally a wimp and if I can do this then they can do it, and I'm here. Support is important, it's really important.

I'm not saying go in with a positive attitude. I would never say that to a client, but with my energy and my voice they can feel it, that cancer's not a death sentence: life goes on. This is just a clink in the machinery, but you fix it and you just move on. I would recommend that you get to know your body, and I tell my students at Colgate that it's important to know your bodies and to recognize any changes. And you know what? It's important to touch yourself. A regular examination isn't a horrible thing. If I hadn't found that lump, my gosh. I had made a donation to the American Cancer Society because of my mother, and with it they sent me this self-exam thing that you hang up in the shower. My daughter didn't want to put it in her shower, so I put it in my shower, and that's when I started examining myself. I thought, oh my, this wasn't there before.

This lump was never picked up in a regular mammogram, and it had been growing in me for ten years. They're now doing MRIs of the breast, which is a very detailed x-ray sort of a thing but they're extremely expensive. My doctor thought I would qualify for a program down in Westchester and so she submitted my name, but I wasn't qualified for it because of my prognosis. Now Bassett is doing MRIs of the breast and I might be qualified for that study. If you don't have a lump, if you don't have something to find in a sonogram, then it won't work. Unfortunately the MRIs are so expensive and they can be used for so many different things. So, get to know your bodies.

I am a mover and things really never kept me down, you know. My first chemo treatment was in the beginning of January on a Monday and that previous Sunday my father had died. I had moved my parents up here from New York to be closer to me because they needed help. So, then I had to have chemo on the Monday after my father died, and we didn't have a funeral until Wednesday. Life goes on. I'm a mover. I've always dealt with pain and dance. You know, you get hurt sometimes. I toss my body, I take risks and move on with it. So I guess those experiences helped me.

You know they say you're okay after five years, but I still get checked every three months. I'm on Tamoxifen, a hormone suppressant, which really only works for five years after you've been diagnosed. I end my Tamoxifen in October, so right now I'm free of cancer. I've known people who have had reoccurrences in their ninth year. Right now I'm good.

And I think this book is going to be very helpful. Hopefully, it will be successful and people will be able to hear the stories and not feel alone if the fact is that they're not ready to talk to people. Maybe they can read about what I've learned. For example, on the first day of chemo I misread the directions on these pills that I was supposed to take four hours before the treatment. I thought you were supposed to take them four hours after the treatment. Oh my God. I came home, I didn't stop puking for two days. It was like it just killed me. It just killed me.

I was asked if there is anything in my background that prepared me for this, and that's a good question. I was the youngest of three children with two older brothers, and I really went through the rigmarole when I was young. My mother and father had me when they were forty-two years old, very old to have children, to have me. My oldest brother is ten years older than I am. They started younger but all they wanted was a daughter with long hair to be a ballerina. They didn't care how long, they were going to try, and here I came along when they were forty-two years old. Growing up on New York City's Lower East Side made me a tough person, and to this day I attribute a lot of that to whom I am now.

A girlfriend of mine who was raised around here won't let her children take trips, and I said when I was eight years old I was already taking the bus and subway to music lessons and to dance lessons all over the city by myself. It's where I was raised and how I was raised. I was raised very independently. My parents were both college professors. I did my thing as a kid. I had my brothers to support me. When I was in seventh grade my parents went to Europe for six months and they left us, my middle brother who was just starting high school and my oldest brother who was just starting college, alone for six months. Yeah, we had a good time. But it was very different. So, you know, I had to toughen it up.

Postscript

"Support is important; it's really important." Like many of the other survivors in this book, Jane found the support of her friends and family extremely important. This support helped Jane to maintain her sense of self and her proactive attitude toward the cancer.

Jane's proactive attitude toward treatment was evident from the start even though her initial reaction was one of shock and anxiety. She did not allow the cancer or the treatments to consume all of her attention or define her as a person. Jane tells us she purposefully focused on things that were more positive so that the cancer would not overwhelm her.

Her behavior protected her sense of self-efficacy. As she continually returned to her normal routine, she minimized the impact of the cancer experience itself, which also contributed to her ability to "get through the experience." Reducing the threat associated with treatment makes the treatment more tolerable.

Jane's story provides us with further evidence of the power and value of social support and the strength of the resilient spirit. Jane's determination to stay focused on "living" contributed to her resilience and provided others with concrete recommendations for coping with health care crises like breast cancer.

Thank you, Jane.

Eleven

Lynne

I was born in Rome, New York and grew up in Floyd, New York. I went to school in Oriskany. I'm the middle child and have an older brother and a younger sister. I have an AAS degree from Cazenovia College in advertising design and a BS in professional and technical communication from SUNYIT. I had just started the IDT program at SUNYIT and then found out I was sick, so I stopped taking classes. I hope I'll get back to them sometime soon. I've been married for twenty years to a great guy.

I was diagnosed in February 2006 and here's why I went to the doctor: I love to antique and I went to an antique show where I bought a painting for $20. I sold it at auction for a lot of money, so that year I had a really great January. After I sold the painting I said, "Well now that I have all this money I want to make sure I'm healthy to enjoy it." So I scheduled my checkups for early February.

My mammogram did not show any cancer but showed a cyst. The technician came in and said the doctor wanted to do a sonogram. The sonogram showed a tumor right next to the cyst. The doctor came into the room and said, "I'm not saying it's cancer, but it might be. What do you want to do?"

I'd never had to deal with this type of thing. I said, "Recommend someone." Later that night, after my brain started to kick in, I called my friends who had had problems and asked them who they'd gone to. They all told me the same doctor's name. I already had an appointment with a different surgeon, but I called my OB/GYN's office and asked them to cancel that appointment and make one with the doctor that my friends and family members recommended. Because I asked around and changed doctors, I was able to have a biopsy a week earlier than I would have. I guess the lesson here is be your own advocate by saying, "No, that's not what I want; I want this."

My cancer was non-hormonal but HER2 positive. Typically you don't know what this means before a diagnosis because you think breast cancer is breast cancer, right? I think the most annoying thing about cancer is that there is no one answer (or cure) for everyone. Because of the size and type of cancer I was diagnosed with I had to do chemotherapy. I call the first round the "evil" chemicals. One of them is red, and to this day I don't consume red Jello or juice—maybe that will change someday. After the evil treatments (and the loss of my hair) I did twelve weeks of a drug called Taxol, and Herceptin, and then had to finish out a year with Herceptin.

My oncologist recommended a standard treatment for the "evil drugs," which was once every three weeks for people with early stage breast cancer. But I decided to go dose-dense—which is biweekly. I said torture me harder for a shorter period of time.

After my initial sadness and anger at the diagnosis, I just started thinking, okay, how do I get through this? One step at a time—and then I came up with the idea of putting everything into phases. Surgery was phase I, chemotherapy phase II, etc., and now that I look back at that year I think wow, that was very hard, but when I segmented it out into little components, it wasn't as bad.

One way of coping in the beginning was to take control over my hair loss. I used to have long hair and even though I'm the type of person who doesn't get her hair done all the time, the hair loss was a big deal. I kept asking the doctor do I have to have chemotherapy and if so, am I going to lose my hair? My hair really started to fall out on May 5, right after my second treatment.

When my husband came home from work that night I asked him to shave my head. He asked, "Are you sure?" He took the buzzer and asked if I wanted to do the first swipe and I said no. He buzzed off all my hair and saved a little bit and the rest he threw out for the birds to put in their nests, and it was gone. The hair had to go, but from now on every May 5, I'm going to drink a toast to that day, my hair, and life.

One thing that really helped me was to visualize my cancer. It's an unknown entity, and I really couldn't grasp it. I don't know how I came up with this, but the night before my surgery, I pictured a big ball of snot inside of me. And then I thought, oh, okay, I've got it now because that way it's disgusting and it needs to be removed. Of course you can see a slide of cancer, but that doesn't really mean much to me.

For the most part, I don't mind talking about cancer, but you start thinking that sometimes people just want to ask because it's polite—when in reality they don't want to know about it because it's a scary thing. Sometimes I'd feel as if I was giving others support versus them giving me support. When people asked how I was doing I'd put it back on them and say, "I'm great; how are you doing?" People are concerned and it's really nice that they're concerned, but after awhile you don't even want to discuss it because you don't want to think about the reality of it all.

I think the medical profession forgets that typically people who have gotten cancer are not in the medical field. We don't know what certain terminologies are, and we don't know initially that we can ask for certain things. I learned pretty quickly that you have to be an advocate for yourself and speak up if you need something.

Another thing a patient may not know is that you don't have to use the recommended doctor. After my initial visit with one of the recommended doctors (a whopping ten minutes with the doctor), I didn't have a good feeling about it. The doctor was also not on my insurance plan. I asked myself why would you want to go to a doctor whom you have to pay out of pocket and who needs a personality adjustment? I found a doctor who was on my plan and who took the time and care to answer all my questions. This doctor is someone I would recommend to others.

Some positive things came from having cancer. My parents bought me this little board to do beading on because I couldn't read; it made me sick to my stomach. So I started stringing beads and made all these ankle bracelets and sold them for $5 each, and I raised $2,000.

We also had a special walk on campus at SUNYIT on the Tuesday before the official Making Strides walk. We had about seventy faculty and staff walk during our lunch hour. Overall, we raised just over $5,000. Before the walk they asked me to say a few words. I thanked everybody for their support and told them it's not about me—it's about trying to come up with a cure so people don't have to go through what I went through. It's too hard.

Postscript

Lynne's attitude and behavior set her up well for a positive recovery. Her response to her cancer diagnosis early on was to take charge of her treatment course, and she tells us, "the lesson here is being your own advocate by saying no, that's not what I want, and I want this."

Lynne also used a number of very good strategies to get through the cancer treatment. For example, she broke the cancer experience into phases so that it would not be so overwhelming or threatening. She says, "when I segmented it out into little components it wasn't as bad."

Lynne also used a number of other strategies to cope with her fears and the cancer. She directly faced her fear of losing her hair by having her husband shave her head. This way Lynne was in control of the hair loss. She determined when and how she was going to shed her hair. An action such as this empowers people in situations where they feel powerless.

Lynne also used visualization to get a "fix" on the cancer. She envisioned the cancer as "disgusting snot." This did two things for Lynne: it gave her a concrete way of dealing with and disposing of the cancer and it made it more "knowable" and therefore less threatening. Lynne tells us, "I pictured a big ball of snot inside of me and then I thought, oh, okay, I've got it now because that way it's disgusting and it needs to be removed."

Both the visualization and the removal of her hair are examples of the proactive, take-charge strategies she used to deal with the reality of breast cancer. Lynne's narrative highlights the strength and resilience of the human spirit. She, like all the other women in this book, provides us with tangible ways for maintaining a sense of self-efficacy in the face of breast cancer.

Thank you, Lynne.

Twelve

Cris

I was born in Utica and lived there until I was about five years old when my family moved to Whitesboro. Now I live approximately a mile and a half from where I grew up, so I haven't gone very far. I did live in New Jersey for two years, where my first child was born. I had one brother who was six years older than me, and sadly my brother passed away from colon cancer at the age of forty-five. My mother is eighty-seven and doing very, very well. I always wanted to be a teacher and I had twenty-seven years of teaching.

Cancer is a major illness in my family. I have had two occurrences of breast cancer. My first diagnosis was four years ago in February. My second diagnosis was, I will not forget, on Halloween of 2006. The cancer was in a different breast the second time, so both are considered primary cancers and unrelated. I have very aggressive forms of cancer. Both of my tumors were fast growing, when compared to some slower growing tumors that take time to develop, so when I was diagnosed it was obvious what to do for both of them. I also had lymph node involvement in both sides, which is important information, so I had lymph nodes removed.

Having cancer the second time was different. When I was diagnosed the first time, I totally curled up in a fetal position on my couch and covered myself with a blanket. That was my initial reaction physically. There are the tears and, of course, the feeling that maybe you're going to die. And I guess I lay there for maybe an hour and got up and ate my dinner and things just started to happen after that. The second time it was more like disappointment, disappointment in my body because I do have a very healthy lifestyle.

I went down to the Dana Farber Cancer Institute in Boston, and I would highly recommend this medical facility. It's an absolutely unbelievable facility. I saw a Harvard medical professor oncology specialist. As a result, what I'm getting this time are drugs from the 1970s, the older chemo protocol for breast cancer. They're different, with fewer side effects.

Everything is a challenge. Cancer itself is a challenge, and I just keep going back to positives and facing that challenge. I used to run away from things that were difficult, but I'm facing this one and it's okay. One of the things that I think is pretty positive about me is that I'm always willing to ask for help, and I'm willing to take suggestions. I have a friend whose husband is a psychiatrist, and I went to him for therapy and learned self-hypnosis, meditation, yoga, and visualization that I used throughout my treatments. It's called integrative medicine. I did self-hypnosis every day before I went to radiation and when I was finished with radiation my doctor said, "Wow you have very little burning!" So for me self-hypnosis is a very powerful experience.

As far as the positives, just this morning I listed ten positives, maybe nine, from having cancer. I'm more self-confident. I always had a belief in God, and I've definitely held on to this and I knew I wasn't going through this by myself. And I have used my creativeness. I took up water color painting, I'm a quilter, and I love to garden.

I think the biggest obstacle is fear. I really learned how to face fear and really walk through fear rather than run away from it. And one of the things I learned was to be an advocate for myself. I ended up changing doctors midstream in my treatment, and it was wonderful. There are some wonderful doctors. I also learned a lot about medicines. The darker these chemo drugs are the more toxic and potent they are. I learned a lot about side effects. Even though chemotherapy is wonderful, there are side effects and some of them are long term.

I think I definitely have become a stronger person, and I probably realize how resilient I am. This strength and resilience were there prior to cancer with other occurrences in my life. So I think having cancer has just upped me even more. Something I can say is that I probably blow myself away.

Postscript

"Everything is a challenge. Cancer is a challenge, and I just keep going back to positives and facing challenges. I used to run away from things that were difficult, but I am facing this one and that's okay." Cris became proactive in the face of two bouts with breast cancer. Her story is inspiring because it illustrates how a person can face a difficult experience and benefit from it at the same time.

Cris used her social support network to seek out help and suggestions. She did not expect others to "fix" the problem; rather Cris listened to advice, evaluated it, and tried out the suggestions. She was open to strategies from integrative medicine where she found techniques that aided her physically and mentally through the experience of breast cancer. She learned to use self-hypnosis, mediation, yoga, and visualization. She reports that self-hypnosis actually resulted in less burning after radiation.

Through Cris's strong faith, she experienced the treatment with a sense of support, and she tells us, "I always had a belief in God, and I've definitely held on to this, and I knew I wasn't going through this myself." These proactive attitudes and behaviors, strong spiritual beliefs, and strategies offered by integrative medicine resulted in

Cris successfully navigating breast cancer treatment and changing for the better as a person.

In a powerful statement, Cris tells us she no longer runs away from fear, but "walks through it." Her sense of self-efficacy increased, as did her creative capacities, which is not unusual following cancer. Sometimes the experience forces people to recognize their strengths and sheds them of the greatest obstacle to creativity and happiness—fear.

Cris's newfound ability to walk through the fear psychologically improved her sense of self-efficacy because she conquered her fear. Cris learned she had power over her fear and so she no longer expended energy trying to avoid it. Her words, "I took up water color painting; I'm a quilter, and I love to garden," reveal that she uses her energies being creative and open to the simple, pleasant experiences of everyday life.

Thank you, Cris.

Thirteen

Jackie

I think I was resilient in my mother's womb. When she was pregnant with me she had fallen and she had a very difficult birth with me and they didn't want to save me; they were just going to save her. We ended up being in the hospital for three weeks, and we both came home December 7, 1941. World War II started then, and my father from that day forward said that I caused World War II, which I actually believed at the time. So I always say I'm resilient from the womb.

My father quit high school at sixteen, but my mother graduated from high school and they got married at seventeen and eighteen and had me at eighteen and nineteen. My mother was a manic depressive from the time I was twelve. I'm the oldest of seven children and the first educated in my family. We lived on the wrong side of the tracks, and I remember five of us living in a three-room apartment with no heat, just a coal stove and a kerosene heater.

I grew up in Liberty, New York, in the Catskills and went to a very small high school. We lived on a farm.

I knew how to run a bulldozer and a bailer at the age of eight and had to drive a thirty-foot truck looking under the wheel. I graduated from Ithaca College and received my master's degree from Syracuse University. I have two master's degrees. I taught high school for thirty-five years in New Hartford. I also raised my three youngest sisters. Whatever you tell me I can't do, I can do. They told me when I got rheumatic fever that I couldn't be a physical education teacher, but I was a physical education teacher. I coached track for thirty-four years, gymnastics for eighteen years, and fall varsity and junior-varsity field hockey for thirty-two years.

Former students really come into play a lot in my life with help for my mother and me. A former student was my radiologist who did the stereotactic biopsy, and she happened to be on vacation so I had to wait until January 6 to have that done. I knew exactly what was going to happen because I had gone through it with my mother. You lie on your stomach with your breast through a hole. The radiologist sits there and cuts.

My mother went through it fine, but I didn't. My tumor was deep in the chest wall so I had to be up on a hip, very uncomfortable. They twisted my neck and my head, and instead of being clamped once I was clamped eight or nine times. I kind of knew it was cancer when they told me the mammogram didn't look normal. The radiologist said it looked suspicious and told me, "If you want to get a jump on this, go home and call Dr. X and see if he can see you right away."

I was diagnosed on Friday, and Monday I saw the first surgeon. The radiologist was so great to me; she gave me her cell phone and we talked about six nights in a row. When I was diagnosed, I didn't cry at all. I was like, go get it. Talking to people was one of my best resources. I did some crying later on, but then I just talked to as many people as I could who'd recently had cancer surgery. A lot of teachers called to tell me that no two cancers are alike. They really aren't. Everybody has something a little bit different.

On Monday one of my sisters, a nurse practitioner, came from Lafayette to go with me to see the first surgeon. I was all set to have him do it; however, I did want a second opinion. So that night I called up a former student who said, "I think I can get you an appointment in Syracuse." She said, "There's this great doctor there; she's not taking any more patients, but maybe you can see one of her associates. She has two or three." She got me in.

I called her Monday night, and on Tuesday at five o'clock, Dr. Newman's office called and said she'd see me the next day at three o'clock. First of all, I didn't have the slides, the biopsies, or the x-rays, and Wednesday was the worst day in Central New York. I called a former student who called to see if the x-rays and the slides would be ready on Wednesday morning at 9:00. I couldn't even walk out of my driveway that day because everything was covered in ice. My neighbor had to drive onto my lawn to pick me up. Then he took me to St. Luke's to get the slides and the x-rays, and then we drove to Syracuse.

It was the twelfth of January. I know the exact date. I was diagnosed on the seventh, I had already been to two surgeons by the twelfth, and this one was not taking any more patients, but I'm very personable and said, "Jeez, you look like you're about my age." She said, "Hey, we were born the same year," and I said, "Oh, that was a good year." We talked like that until she was done. The two opinions were very different. If they had been the same I would've gone with the local person. I asked her, "Would you consider taking me as another patient, please?" She said, "Oh sure," so I gave her a hug and a kiss.

The experience had some positive results: I got closer to God, really, a lot closer. I had a lot of different little obstacles along the way. I handled everything beautifully, I think, until I hit radiation. Before I was diagnosed with cancer, I'd had weakness in my midsection for two years. I'm a physical education teacher, but I couldn't get out of a chair without using my arms, and I'd collapse when I'd sit. It started two years ago and got worse this past summer, so I started seeing a neurologist in the fall. I went through tests all fall, like EMGs. Then I had an MRI of the brain because they thought I had Multiple Sclerosis.

Then in November one of my best friends, who is

about twelve years younger, was diagnosed with inoperable lung cancer. All this happened in November. I went for the mammogram and then throughout the process little obstacles came up, like when I went for an echogram the Wednesday before surgery and found out I have a leaky heart valve. Then they said, "We don't know if we're going to operate." But the next day I went for a stress test, and afterwards they said, "You've got the heart of a horse, just a leaky valve."

A lot of other little obstacles also came up down the road. The needle localization was horrible. The easiest part was the surgery. I went home the same day, late at night, but I couldn't drive for a week. I live alone, but I have four sisters, and each of them stayed a day with me. You're sent home with a drain because there's this pocket. I walked a lap the first morning, and the second day I started my exercises, so I did well. A week later I was swimming, and twelve days later I was playing tennis. When I went to have my stitches out, the surgeon told me I might have to have chemo and my tumor was on the borderline. She said it'd be interesting to see what the oncologist said.

When I drove to Syracuse again to see the oncologist, she found a lump between my two scars. She didn't tell me what to do. She said I had a choice. You want to be told what to do. It was like she kind of recommended that I not have the chemo because of this other thing that I have going on with polyneuropathy and stuff. I was upset because she didn't tell me what to do.

The next day I had to go back to get the tumor checked. I had decided not to have the chemo at that point. I talked to the nurse practitioner, and she thought the lump was nothing except that it needed to be drained more. That afternoon I had to go see the radiologist, who said, "You're not having chemo? You've got to get a second or third opinion on whether you're having chemo." I cried then.

On Saturday night a former teacher called me from New Hartford. She'd had breast cancer and bone cancer and cancer that had metastasized in her ribs. She had been to the Dana Farber Cancer Institute three times. She said, "You know Tom Ryan in New Hartford is the smartest guy of anybody I know and he was my mother's oncologist, too." I had taught his kids in school. On Sunday after church I called him, and when his wife answered I gave her my name and said "Barb, I don't know if you remember me but I taught at New Hartford." She said, "Oh yeah, Valerie drove you nuts" and asked me how I was. I said, "Well, I've had a pretty bad weekend." She gave the phone to Tom, and right then he offered to see me Monday morning at 8:00 to sign papers and have my files faxed to his office.

I was there at 7:45 a.m., and they said, "Go back home and come back at 11:00 and he'll see you." University Hospital hadn't faxed any of that stuff. It was finally faxed that afternoon, and I went in to see him Tuesday. His opinion was the same as the other oncologist. He didn't think I needed chemo, so I went with that.

Normally, I go to Florida for a month in February, but the day I was supposed to leave I had surgery. Instead, I made reservations to go for just a week. I went, even though I was still pretty weak, and then started radiation just this previous March 2. I recently finished treatments, and I'm still pretty tired.

Postscript

Jackie tells us that she is resilient and has been since the day she was born! Despite the complications and obstacles encountered, Jackie still maintained a proactive attitude toward her treatment. She sought out the advice of people she trusted and was able to secure the treatment advice she needed. This is certainly an example of resiliency in the face of a difficult treatment course. Jackie never once gave up; she simply kept going and focused on one aspect of the treatment course at a time. No doubt, this helped her tolerate its unpleasant aspects.

The emotional and instrumental support she received from former students and family enhanced Jackie's proactive attitude. Her former students were willing and eager to assist her in any way they could. No doubt this was a reflection of the respect Jackie earned over the years as a teacher and a coach. Sometimes we do reap what we sow, and in Jackie's case, the support from family and friends was well earned. However, Jackie had to accept that support for it to benefit her. Not only did Jackie accept the help, advice, and encouragement received from her supporters, she embraced it. This too is a characteristic of a resilient personality. Resilient individuals know how to get and use the social supports that surround them.

Thank you, Jackie.

About the Authors

Joanne M. Joseph, Ph.D., is Associate Professor of Psychology at SUNY Institute of Technology, Utica, New York where she teaches courses in psychology. She is the author of a number of scholarly publications including the book, *The Resilient Child: Preparing Today's Youth for Tomorrow's World* (Da Capo Press, 2001). Dr. Joseph is a licensed psychologist and regularly provides consultative services to area schools, hospitals, and community agencies. She is the recipient of the Chancellor's Award for Excellence in Teaching and the Chancellor's Award for Excellence in Faculty Service.

Dr. Joseph resides with her husband, Michael Moore, in Clinton, New York. The couple has three children, Catherine, Jessica, and Alexander.

Patricia Murphy, D.A., is an Assistant Professor of English and the Writing Program Coordinator at the SUNY Institute of Technology, Utica, New York. She has authored articles about service-learning and composition pedagogy and has seen publication of her creative work in several literary magazines.

Dr. Murphy is proud to be the daughter of Vincent and Catherine Murphy and mother to Alicia and Catherine Billman. She lives in Clinton, New York.